The Mindfulness of Slowing Down

Improving Health, Wealth, and Joy Through Slow Mindful Movements

Healthy Habits

Thanks for Reading

Table of Contents

Slowing Down Requires Being Mindful

The idea of mindfulness was traditionally used by the followers of Gautama Buddha. In their perception, it was a part of a spiritual journey, something as essential as it is mystical. A mindful approach to life is extremely important for those who profess Buddhism, leading to their ideal of becoming a happy and peaceful person.

Today there is a lot of talking about mindfulness. A lot of people are interested in it, from psychologies and business coaches to political leaders. Dictionaries offer different definitions on "mindfulness," but all of them share one idea, an idea of concentrating your mind and attention on the current moment and experience.

Why is mindfulness worth practicing? For some time, scientists involved in mindfulness research have reported that a habit of mindful thinking leads to positive changes in your brain. Hence, it's a chance to raise your life to a higher level.

This ability of the brain to improve and restructure during a lifetime due to new experience is called neuroplasticity. This notion was mentioned in "The Principles of Psychology" by William James, a psychologist who lived in the second half of 19th century.

Contemporary management professionals believe that this method of thinking provides you with great inner potential. Practicing mindfulness helps to develop a leader's qualities; staying self-confident, calm, merciful, emotionally secure, yet resilient. Nowadays, when almost no one can be sure what is waiting for them tomorrow, mindful leaders are especially needed.

Bill George, one of the leading management insiders, is sure that such rulers can achieve way more than those who are violent and short-tempered. The leaders that are into the idea of mindfulness tend to inspire people rather than to command them. They hear and understand other points of view, know how to behave in stressful situations, and how to cope with crisis.

Most people living today are under an enormous amount of pressure on a daily basis while trying to live their lives in a changeable and often aggressive environment. They have to deal with problems, new situations, and other people who have their own issues. So, that's quite a stressful struggle. It's reasonable to suppose that if mindful thinking can ease our lives, cure our minds, and open the door to a new vision of the world around us, it's worth learning.

Seizing the Moment

Let's see what an experience of mindful thinking can look like. The following information is based on a session with a Buddhist monk who has over 36-years of experience practicing mindfulness named Bhante Wimala.

The ability to live in the moment is essential for keeping your inner energy balanced and being protected from sufferings caused by ups and downs. It doesn't exclude thinking about the future and solving existing problems, but it means focusing on current processes without getting lost in thoughts that are not related to the activity you are involved in at the moment.

According to Zen monks, the road to mindfulness begins with cleaning. Cleaning rituals, including sweeping, raking, dusting, and others, are very important spiritual rituals. The monks think of nothing while cleaning up space, focusing solely on what they are doing. This practice may be followed at home. We all spend some time on housework, so try use this time for your benefit.

How can it be done? Forget about everything else except the moment you are in, notice every detail: how the dust is raising up, how is the fiber by touch, what is the sound of the water falling in a sink. Housework can be turned from a boring duty into the way of mental improvement. Use this tool a couple of times a week or according to your cleaning schedule.

The Fear of Change

Fear is a natural feeling that is familiar to everyone. It is an arm of an organism to protect us from danger. We feel fear and get prepared for coping with some trouble or choose to escape it. It has a crucial meaning for our existence, saving us from danger.

Fear also has an opposite side that is not as pleasant and useful: fear often doesn't let us make our life brighter and more interesting, it stands between new acquaintances and us, between our talents and our self-realization. So, fear is one of the main reasons why we can't move forward sometimes. Emotional pain works the same way, regardless of if it was caused by others or by our own deeds.

A physiological reaction to some kind of threat to survival, and, consequently, to experiencing pain or fear, is called "fight or flight." Mindfulness is an opposite notion, as its main idea is letting go. Such an approach frees our mind from attempting to resist these emotions. As a result, the mind becomes clear.

According to Buddhism philosophy, the more one is connected to a negative feeling, the more suffering he starts to experience. So, it is important to break the bond between you, fear, and pain. We must detach from them, and only then will we have a chance to become free.

What is letting go about, in fact? It's about not judging people around their actions and life choice. It's about learning to forgive and forget and saying "no" to blaming yourself for mistakes and roads taken. Being able to let people, fear, and anger go, underlies one's inner changing and leads to becoming a more flexible and open-minded person. This trip is tough and takes time yet shows a new reality which you never could see before.

Speed Reduction

Today we are so used to always running to get and achieve something, that we do not even realize that there can be another path. It may sound crazy, but to move forward, we need to slow down sometimes. A decision to slow down may open your eyes to the magic of every moment, help you see life under the new light and add positivity to your way of perceiving things.

To make the first step towards a mindful existence, one is not obliged to go out of town for a couple of weeks or become completely isolated. Mindfulness demands a little practice every day without having to leave your normal environment. Slowing down means focusing on one thing that you do or think about without trying to go multi-tasking and get everything done. Doing one activity at a time, staying calm, attentive, and completely involved in it.

Physiology Does Matter

Have you ever noticed when your heart beats faster and when it slows down? It beats slower when you are lying, sitting or standing, and raises its speed when you start to move. Stress also makes a heart run faster, and the tenser the situation is, the faster its rhythm is. Staying calm and relaxed is obviously good for your heart and physical condition in general, as it has been proved that those with fast resting heart rates have a huge risk of high blood pressure. Besides, there is a link with developing sudden death, cardiovascular disease, and atherosclerosis.

The reason why it happens is simple. Artery walls experience stress with every pulse of blood, so a faster heart beat brings a lot of suffering to them, causing their damaging and wearing out. Also, the coronary arteries can't fill with blood like they are supposed to, and heart cells don't get enough oxygen. Obviously, that's not good for health.

There is a way to calm down your heart rate and keep it slow enough, it's a chance to significantly lower the opportunity of getting some form of heart disease. Studies show that exercising more and reducing stressful work is good for your heart even if you previously were among many people with high resting heart rates.

Rare and unbalance physical activity makes your heart beat faster, but if you devote some time exercising from day to day, it helps to slow your heart down. Complement training with medication and anti-stress practices and your heart will be grateful.

Slowing Down Eating

You may have already heard that slow eating is better than fast eating. Some of us have known this since childhood, some found it out when they were already adults. When you are young, advice to spend more than 15 minutes eating is likely to make you irritated, because there are so many things to devote yourself to other than putting food in your mouth. But there are a bunch of good reasons to eat slowly. Proper nutrition and the right way of eating are excellent for both your mind and body.

So, What Will Happen if You Slow Down While Eating?

You'll eat less. At the beginning of 2014 one of the leading medical magazines revealed that when one eats slowly, he is likely to get fewer calories. What's more interesting, there were two groups of people involved in the study. The first one, of those whose weight is considered normal, consumed 88 fewer calories after slowing their eating speed.

The overweight group also showed good results. They got 58 fewer calories. In addition, both groups drank more water when they slowed down, and their appetites were more satisfied. The other study's results demonstrated that the more chews you make, the less food you consume during one meal. Of course, it needs time. And so, we're back to slow eating.

Your Waistline Gets Thinner

Thanks to changing biochemical processes caused by new eating habits, the risk of overeating goes down.

How can all these benefits happen only after you start eating slowly? Let's see. If you consume your food quickly, your body can hardly send all the natural signals to the brain, because it simply doesn't have enough time.

This misbalance influences important natural processes and influences the workings of different systems. There are special hormones that give a signal when we are full, and these hormones are produced during the process of eating.

Ghrelin, the "hunger hormone," and leptin (it's produced by fat cells) are the leading influencers here. Ghrelin appears as an automatic answer of pleasure centers in the brain to consuming food (by the way, the lack of sleep increases production of ghrelin); leptin works to prevent overeating.

Hormones need some time to deliver their message to the brain. Scientists say that it takes 20 minutes on average to complete this process. We should consider that some people suffer from leptin resistance. Hence their brains are not able to receive the signals on time or don't receive them at all. Leptin just needs some time to finish its mission.

So, the truth is simple: if we eat fast, hormones don't have time to do their work, we consume more food than we need, and don't hear our brain which could stop us from getting extra calories. Exercise and choosing healthy food is no less important, but just the way you eat can change a lot in how you look.

The chewing process itself is also more complicated than it may seem. Chewing is essential for right digestion, as it prepares food to go through the digestive tract. The mouth is where fat and carbohydrate transformation begins. Chewing is the first process to start the secretion of hormones, it also activates taste receptors and helps the stomach to secrete hydrochloric acid.

Besides, chewing is a good practice for your jaw and teeth, making them stronger and preventing tooth decay and other problems. And, finally, chewing stops some kinds of bacteria from getting into your gut. If these bacteria enter your organism, you may experience diarrhea, bloating, gas, and other uncomfortable circumstances.

If food is properly chewed, all the nutrients can be easily absorbed in the intestines. But when one swallows his meal instead of measured chewing, food is not prepared for digestion, and so most of the beneficial nutrients leave your body unutilized.

All the nutrients which could make your body healthier and stronger are simply being thrown away. And when your body doesn't get enough necessary nutritious fuel, it sends signals to the brain to eat more regardless of whether you have already finished your portion. Such a false signal leads to gaining extra pounds.

How many chewing motions should we make to get the desirable result? That is a really important question. It is believed that modern people tend to reduce the average number of chews. Partly because we now eat more processed food than ever, choosing it over whole products.

So, if you start consuming raw food, you'll automatically chew more. The opinion on how many chews we should make for every bite differs. Some scientists say it should be no less than 40, while the author of "The Great Masticator" and chewing guru Horace Fletcher offers to make about 100 chewing motions.

A hundred sounds inconvenient and, let's speak the truth, a bit insane. After all, the best choice is to spend as much time chewing every bite as it continues to be comfortable for you. One thing that is useful to know is the perfect moment to swallow. This is when food loses its texture and begins to become liquid.

If you are still not quite sure about whether it is reasonable to change your chewing habits, maybe a chance to return your jaw into its proper shape will interest you. Research shows that chewing will train jaw muscles, so it is good for both your health and appearance. However, you may feel strange and even tired during the first days of your new chewing life, but getting used to it doesn't take a lot of time. A new taste for regular food and reduced portions (because you'll feel full quicker) is a bonus.

The Way to Mindful Eating

All the techniques mentioned above are a part of mindful eating. It's a kind of a movement that perceives eating food as a religious experience. More and more people turn to this philosophy, and even some of the leading world organization are not an exception. Among them Google, which announced that its employees will now have an hour a month devoted to mindful eating.

As an idea of mindfulness, mindful eating also was born thanks to the wise Buddhist monks. They considered eating to be one of the best meditation practices along with standing, silently walking, and cleaning up. The pleasure we get while leisurely consuming food is very important, they believed.

Currently, mindful eating is a popular theme to discuss and to write about. Dr. Jan Chozen Bays, for example, reckons that unconsciousness while eating is a pest of modern society. We are used to combining having a meal with surfing the net, watching TV, texting, or sitting on the phone.

Chozen seems to be right, and that's not surprising, as Dr. Bays also wrote a book about mindful eating. According to the doctor and the Buddhists, your thoughts while you are eating mean no less that what food you are putting in your mouth. Tune inward, focus on what you are eating and where is it from. Try to think of all the people and animals involved in the producing of your meal. Thank them for their time, care, and energy. Slow, silent, thoughtful eating is one of the best ways to meditate and benefit your body and spirit. It is affordable to almost everyone today.

Slowing Down Our Breathing

Breathing is so natural that we usually don't think of this process at all. However, it's also worth our careful attention. We are all born with an ability to breathe with a full chest, we are just so used to it, that sometimes even don't notice when the way we breath starts to change.

According to wellness guru and journalist Don Campbell, there is a whole complex of factors that influence our breathing in a bad way. Among them are, of course, smoking which affects our respiratory system, lack of physical activity, permanent stress, various heart diseases, and a sedentary lifestyle.

Environmental pollution also makes this increase. All these factors don't let us practice our normal breathing, resulting in many sad consequences. As an answer to this situation, a new movement was born, called "conscious breathing." There is good reason for this movement. The average adult living in western society is said to make about 15 breaths per minute. This means that they are using only one-third of their natural lung capacity.

Breathing is one of our basic functions which transformed with evolution. People used to spend their days hunting, raising cattle, working with their hands, often outdoors and regardless of the weather conditions. That lifestyle demanded using their diaphragm to the maximum extent.

However, times changed and the technical progress of the 20th century let many people forget about energy-intensive manual labor. We moved to office spaces, got cars and public transportation. Everything needed for a comfortable, careless, and lazy life. So, there's no wonder that today lung muscles are not used as they could be, and that affects our standard of living.

Don Campbell studied yoga and other physical practices, and in the course of time he found out that 10 slow and deep breaths in a minute work best for our health. One can make even less than 10, as then the parasympathetic nervous system is engaged. And this system does a lot in healing the body if there is any injury.

While breathing slowly, one provides their lungs' cells with enough oxygen. It helps the body to relax. This fact is supported by doctors. For example, Dr. Fred Muench. His company, Mobile Health Interventions, created a new iOS app, which tracks your breathing and tells what breathing rates are optimal for your body. As a result, a user has a chance to rearrange his breathing and become more energetic and concentrated.

Alpha waves in the brain increase thanks to slow breathing, which are really good for our ability to think clearly. There is one more benefit: slow breathing makes our heart rate during certain kinds of activity more variable, which is naturally healthier than a stable one.

For example, if one's heart beats between 65 and 85 times per minute, it's more advantageous for their health than if the heart rate runs between 70 and 75 beats. A small heart-rate usually characterizes quite an old person or somebody with health issues, while significant heart swings are seen among athletes and fit people. The good news: we can improve our heart's variability by learning to breathe slowly.

Campbell says that they experimented with plenty of ways to slow breathing down, but one of them appeared to be the most effective. He doesn't see any necessity to breathe slowly all the time and advises to practice it just 5 or 6 times daily.

One of his followers reports that his body and mind experienced significant changes after he developed this habit. Among them, he names improving energy levels, mental focus, creativity, and concentration. This also resulted in the healing of his neck and shoulder zones which previously brought him some suffering.

So, let's see what relearning how to breathe means. A lot of people don't use the diaphragm fully, and this exercise is aimed to rearrange it. Firstly, inhale deeply, then exhale as you want to blow out a candle (with a short burst).

Exhale slowly to leave your lungs empty. Make a slow uninterrupted breath, trying to feel the lungs from the bottom to the top. Wait a few seconds as oxygen needs a little time to saturate your cells. Then exhale completely, and of course, slowly. To finish the exercise, repeatedly go through these steps for 5 minutes.

Slowing Down Our Work Life

Workers of the 21st century experience huge pressures despite technological innovations in many industries existing today. People work hard and are physically and emotionally exhausted. They must do different tasks at one time, control a lot of things, and they don't even take enough breaks to rest and relax. And, what is the most interesting, their productiveness often doesn't increase at all. Instead, it tends to get lower as the amount of duties gets higher.

Productivity is worth worrying about. No matter how many digital supportive tools a worker can use, if he is stressed and overloaded with tasks (all of them, of course, are urgent to carry out), the results will leave much to be desired. Americans studies of labor demonstrate that hourly output per worker went down in 2015 compared with 2014.

We should also consider such effects of hard work on physical and mental health issues. There are studies which notify that more than 55 working hours per week may lead to depression, diabetes, and heart illnesses.

So, there's no surprise that there is a significant demand for meditation practices and other branches of a mindfulness lifestyle. By the way, this industry is today estimated at about $1 billion. Slowing down may be the only reasonable way to fix up your career, health, and life. Just another reason to look at what the benefits slowing down may bring you.

Realizing There is Enough Time

How often do you think that you are short on time? Let us suppose that happens often. Too often. Maybe always. Living in such a state of mind causes plenty of stress and suffering. Of course, planning to get more and achieve more is not a bad idea and can make your life brighter. But this way of thinking and living may cause more damage than success.

Instead, "slow" thinking as a cognitive state seems to appear way more advantageous. This style of thinking provides you with creativity, intuition, insights, and breakthroughs. When your mind breaks free from pressure, it starts to produce new ideas like never before. The experience of slow thinking helps to avoid getting furious at work, quickly switching between unfinished tasks, an exhausting schedule, and a large portion of stress. Productivity improves when we have a strong ability to focus on one activity at a time, and slowing down teaches us how to do it without any worries or need for multi-tasking.

Slowing Down Our Thinking

According to "Thinking, Fast and Slow" (by Daniel Kahneman), our mind can work in two modes. The first way of thinking exists thanks to the sympathetic nervous system; it is automatic, fast, and is similar to a survival instinct. The second one is based on the parasympathetic nervous system; it is more slow, logical, and rational. In his book, Kahneman draws our attention to the importance of the interconnection between these states of mind.

According to him, out way of thinking forms our views, decisions, and choices in every sphere of life, from business to leisure time. The author writes about the ability of slow thinking to push forward our mental boundaries. This doesn't mean we no longer need a logical part. But slow thinking provides us with the time and opportunity to listen to our intuition, to see the situation from all its angles, to calmly draw conclusions. It's a fact that if one has enough time to think, he's more likely to come to the best possible decision.

Learning to listen

Having a chance to finish your monolog without being interrupted can be named a real asset today. However, interruptions are very common. Such a habit is not only unethical and impolite, but it also depreciates the communication process, making it ineffective and unsatisfying.

Communication can bring us so much joy! To make this happen, we need to learn to listen to each other. If you slow down and draw attention to what a person in front of you is talking about, what is his position, what's on his mind, what he is worried about, you may discover something very special. The chance of misunderstanding each other also goes down then.

Correcting your Mistakes to Escape Repeating Them

As already mentioned, multi-tasking doesn't turn you into a more productive person. Instead, is causes a lot of messy mistakes and missteps that irretrievably devour your time and energy like a black hole. Trying to cope with several tasks at a time leads to working inefficiently, damages brain resources, and puts you under enormous stressful pressure. After all is said and done, you will spend hours coping with the sad results of multi-tasking.

When we switch from new tasks to correcting old ones and back, we end up with memory issues and a bunch of unfinished or poorly done tasks. The brain can't differ truly important activities from those that can wait, so its potential is often wasted for nothing. But slowing down helps a lot here. When we do things one after another, staying calm and concentrated on the current process, it is way easier to notice every little detail and prevent unwanted circumstances. If we slow down, our mind focuses on things of primary importance and maintains its energetic level. Slowing down leads to efficient work.

Teaching our Brains the Habit of Slowing Down

The brain is a wonderful organ that has an outstanding ability to transform itself as a response to life experiences. So, when we start to change our lifestyle, the brain adapts to it and begins to function on a new level. The thing is we just need to trigger this process and make some efforts in the beginning, but then our brains will continue changing on their own.

That is why meditation practices do have a positive effect on our mental health and potential. Some studies show that the brains of those who are advanced meditators are likely to be better preserved than of those who are not interested in meditation.

Meditation is great for teaching our brain to be able to pause before acting. Daniel Siegel, the psychiatrist, named this skill "response flexibility." It helps us to avoid impulsiveness by becoming more flexible in taking decisions and responding to signals, situations, and circumstances.

So, a good level of mental energy, an ability to focus and take your time, and avoiding mistakes, are the skills of an attentive listener – these and other effects of mindfulness will obviously make you a more productive, perspective, and healthy worker.

9 Tips for Slowing Down

Technological progress was meant to save the time and resources of humanity, but nevertheless, people chose to find more and more things to do instead. We are still in a time trap, trying to catch every opportunity, emotion, and experience. Life has turned out to be so fast and impetuous, that one can easily miss his chance to enjoy it. The obvious answer to how to seize the beauty of the moment is slowing down.

Are you tired of the regular rush off to your workspace? Do you want to forget about these nervous moments? Have you ever thought about how much time you spend connected to your gadgets? Exhausted of multi-tasking? Then it's time to slow down and learn how to enjoy every minute of your life. It's a conscious choice, leading to an appreciation of our days and the world around us by opening our hearts to happiness. Slowing down requires some efforts, especially in the beginning of the journey, but the recommendations are quite simple.

Here and Now

Focusing on your current moment is an ability of primary importance. Learning to bring your thoughts back to the present will benefit your mind and level of satisfaction with life. Notice when you analyze your past or feel nostalgic about it, dream of the future too much, or try to guess what else might happen to you or someone else. If noticed, pull yourself together and return to the present moment. Being here and now, concentrated on what you are doing and your environment, means a lot.

Say No to Multi-Tasking

You need to analyze your plans and decide what needs to be done right now. When decided, concentrate on it until you are finished. Remember, focusing on a single task at a time is way more efficient and saves you energy. Leave some space between tasks in your daily schedule. If so, you'll have time to enjoy the things that bring you joy.

Be Close to Nature

Today this perfect source of strength, energy, inspiration, and calmness is so often ignored by citizens who prefer to be prisoned inside their homes, offices, and vehicles. But walking outdoors and observing nature is necessary for our inner harmony. Breathing fresh air, watching water and greenery, listening to rustling leaves helps to maintain the mental balance. There is a wide choice of what you can do outdoors, beginning with doing sports, exercising and hiking to walking in a park. Your personal daily meetings with nature are essential for mindful living.

Put Aside our Gadgets

Most people got so used to their cell phones, tablet computers, and other mobile devices that they can hardly endure even an hour without scrolling and texting. Of course, that is no good. Practice disconnecting from your digital part of life from time to time. Switch off your phone or don't take it with you whenever it is possible.

Do pauses while working on a computer and turn to other things for a while. Being always connected means that you are always interrupted by others, getting messages, and are tempted to open Instagram or something technological. Slowing down is only possible when your mind is in the "real" reality, not in the digital one.

Connect

Have you ever thought of how you spend time with your friends, relatives, colleagues, and loved ones? Often communicating with people is not as close and sincere as it could be. This happens due to various reasons. We are focused on ourselves and our problems, distracted by the phone, analyzing work issues and so on.

We often don't even really think of a person in front of us. It's like you have some automatic mode for meetings. But slowing down means, above all, close connections with people who you love, respect, and admire. Talk to them, think about them, emphasize them, be truly involved, and your relationship will raise to the next level.

Slow Down our Car

A fast-paced world's habits include speedy driving that causes wasting of fuel, traffic accidents and a whole bunch of negative energy that is familiar to almost every driver. But there's no big sense in it.

Au contraire, slower driving gives a chance to enjoy the view, avoid stress, and it's much safer. Slow driving means taking care of yourself and your passengers. It gives you a feeling of control and calmness.

Breath Practices

Breathing is a perfect way to cope with stressful situations quickly, and it also helps to seize the moment. Take a deep breath, then a couple more. When fresh air fills your lungs, stress leaves your body. Focus on your breath to relax or slow down: slowly inhale, exhale, inhale, exhale.

Talk Slow

Fast and loud speech patterns often raise the feelings of stress. Try to carry out a small experiment: while you are in a company of fast or loud talking friends (or other people), switch to slow calm talking, making pauses. Your companions may unconsciously adapt to new speaking and support it. If not, don't worry!

You now have a chance to feel free from speed, anxiety, and aggression, and can look at the situation from a small distance. Just try not to fall for these speedy loud moods again. Stay strong and calm.

Personal Pleasures

It's a new step on your way to the art of being here and now. Learn to find something positive and pleasant in every action you are involved in. Smells, noises, rhythms, emotions – find your own way to pleasure.

For example, while washing the dishes you may be surprised by how graciously the water falls, and the whole task will appear to be way more satisfying. Life is full of surprises and things to enjoy; it is just waiting for you to open your eyes and mind to find them.

What are the Results of Slowing Down?

You'll begin to look at the environment in a new light, instead of continuing this permanent rush. You'll realize who you are, what are your feelings and emotions, where are you, and who are you surrounded by. You will analyze the priorities and find out what is meaningful and urgent for you.

Your mind will experience a new level of energy, concentration, productiveness, and clearness. You will feel inner harmony and calmness that you can share with the world. Slowing down prevents you from losing yourself in an illusionary reality and switching between the past and the future. Freedom and happiness will arise instead of worries and that is what slowing down is about.

www.ingramcontent.com/pod-product-compliance
Lightning Source LLC
Chambersburg PA
CBHW051404280526
45784CB00007B/3090